THE BEFEFITS OF ACUPUNCTURE

Treatment for Fertility, Depression, Weight Loss and More.

By Sally Pederson

Thank you for purchasing this book. Please review
this book on Amazon. I need your feedback so I can
make the next version even better. Thank you very
much.

For other books by this author go to:
https://www.amazon.com/author/sallypederson

Table of Contents

Introduction

All forms of life in this world owe their existence to a particular force which is aptly named as life force. While through its presence this force ensures the existence of life, its absence is the sure sign of death, thus emphasizing its importance.

Thousands of years ago, people in China realized the vitality of this life force not just for the sake of ensuring life but also health. Having named it as 'Qi' they plotted the pathways through which it flowed through the body and prepared charts depicting its motion. Based on this learning they realized that any disruption in its pathway led to ill-health and that this obstacle could be successfully overcome by inserting sharp implements at certain points along the body. Over a period of time a needle began to be favored as instruments to carry out this technique and thus was born acupuncture, the ancient Chinese method of treating medical conditions.

Known to be effective against a wide array of illnesses ranging from liver malfunctioning to stress and chronic pain, acupuncture entails inserting needles at certain critical points on the skin of the patient and these are referred to as acupoints. More often than not, these are totally unrelated to the area of disorder but their main function is to dissolve the obstacles that hinder the flow of 'Qi'. Thus, the aim of the acupuncturist is to trigger acupoints so that the flow of Qi along its meridians is restored and stimulated and the healing process of the body is set into motion. In this way, various problems, whether these are physical ailments, problems like drugs and alcohol, mental issues or pregnancy can be treated irrespective of the age and gender of the person.

Like all physicians, even the acupuncturist relies on certain tools to make his diagnosis. However, the similarity ends there because the tools used in acupuncture originate in nature namely the five elements and Yin and Yang. Fire, earth, water, wood and metal are the five elements into which are internal organs are classified into and it is the aim of the acupuncturist which of the five elements requires to be attended to. All five of these elements are linked to seasons as well which why people often experience health problems during seasonal changes. Yin and yang is a pair that is representative of opposites – while the former reflects calmness and cool, the latter is indicative of excess heat and strong emotions. For a body to enjoy good health balance between the yin and yang is a must and this is what is ensured by the acupuncturist.

Traditionally hailing from china, acupuncture as a mode of treatment arrived in Europe during the 1700s' and subsequently it arrived in America. Some of the reasons which added to its popularity in these parts of the world are its non-invasive nature, lack of side effects and its efficacy. Of course, selection of an acupuncturist is something that should never be overlooked and efforts should be made to identify one who seems to be most compatible with the patient.

Acupuncture: An Overview

Credit goes to the Chinese for having developed and used acupuncture in treatment since many centuries. In China it is a traditional method of curing and is known as Zhue Jiao, meaning "needle heat". It is based on the concept that the human body comprises of an inner energy known as Qi. The needles control this energy in a bid to restore physical health, relieve stress and control mental health.

When at the epitome of health, any individual should have free flowing Qi energy so as to remain well balanced, keeping everything the cells need for maintenance in check and removing waste. This balance is essential for maintaining physical and mental health in good order. If Qi is stopped, the body experiences illness and the acupuncturist needs to determine where the needles need to be placed in order to bring the flow back to normal. Depending on the severity, treatment could happen during one sitting or may require several sessions. Chinese get acupuncture as often as possible to maintain good heath. Likewise, the practitioner gets paid only if a client remains healthy.

Though all techniques of acupuncture rely on needles, there are certain variations, such as electric stimulation, burning and incorporation of herbs. In sharp contrast to those used in Western medicine, Chinese needles are solid. Pre-sterilized and disposable needles are used by acupuncture practitioners in America. No medication is used on the needle, because the needle by itself acts on Qi energy and changes the flow. The practitioner might rotate or manipulate the needle a little or use a certain angle to insert it if he feels that it would have a positive impact on the patient's body.

A particular problem related to physical health or an unsettling emotion to be addressed may need just one or two visits or a series of visits to obtain positive results. This greatly depends on the extent of the problem. The acupuncturist may insert several needles during a visit and during subsequent visits the locations for the needles may be changed as the condition improves.

Needles are inserted just beneath the layer of skin and at times these may be inserted up to the depth of three inches of the epidermis. There is an occasional tingling feeling when the needle is inserted and sometimes there is a warm and relaxing sensation accompanying the insertion of needles around the point of insertion. This is an indication that the Qi flow is properly coordinated and is on its way to normalcy. Once in place, the needles can be forgotten as there is no pain or any sensation surrounding the area.

Regular acupuncture helps maintaining good health and has proven its worth in treating many medical conditions. There are insurance companies offering cover for acupuncture and hence the possibility of using acupuncture could be explored at leisure. After all, what could be a better way of dealing with the problem than addressing its root cause and empowering the body to heal itself from within?

Evolution of Acupuncture

The earliest record for the use of acupuncture has been dated to the reign of the Yellow Emperor in China around 2600 BC. In itself this fact is witness to the theory that Chinese medicine came into existence thousands of years ago.

In the absence of advanced medical facilities which are readily available nowadays, the ancient Chinese noticed that when suffering from a certain health problem, some areas of the skin were more sensitive. Based on this observation they began to record the location of these sensitive areas that dealt with a symptom or the set of symptoms which manifested at that particular point of time. These areas were then associated with the internal organs that were thought to malfunction and cause the illness. An outline of the human body was then drawn and the sensitive points connected in order to explain the function of the entire body in terms of organs.

There were a number of spots marked within this outline of the human body to indicate the sensitive areas. Lines or meridians were then drawn to show the connection between the organs, thereby indicating the energy flow from one organ to the other. It was on the basis of these diagrams and related texts that the concept of energy or Qi being central to the use of acupuncture emerged. As per Chinese literature, all human beings are born with a certain amount of Qi. This degenerates by "living" and is reinstated by food eaten and air inhaled. The imbalance of this Qi at a certain point in life is what gives rise to poor health and its absence means death. Qi moves throughout the body, from meridian to meridian and organ to organ, degenerated and reinstated at every junction.

Needles used in acupuncture affect the energy level or Qi, and this in turn affects organ function by reducing or stimulating it. Some organs such as the liver give a quick and direct response as compared to other organs. Acupuncture can be used for relief from pain, stress and various other symptoms and conditions simply by controlling the energy flow.

Although it was in China that acupuncture as a form of treatment was founded, it is popular amongst the Japanese too who have developed their own techniques of applying this concept. Thus Japanese acupuncture has been derived from its Chinese counterpart, but with its own differences. Acupuncture was introduced in Europe by the Jesuit missionaries who had lived in Beijing during the seventeenth century and even though it was not accepted at that time, there were physicians who practiced it. Many writings on the subject were published by M. Mont, a Frenchman during the 1940s and it was these that sparked the beginning of interest in acupuncture amongst the Western physicians. They began regarding it seriously for the control of pain.

In this contemporary era it is used by physicians in the western world to control pain and relieve stress. For some surgeries no anaesthesia is administered and instead acupuncture is given, the advantage being that patients' organs are not affected by anaesthesia. The interest in acupuncture in the western world has caused people to take an interest in China, where it all began. This in turn has led to the discovery of texts based on acupuncture that have been hitherto unknown. Since these have never been read before, people are looking forward to interpret and expand them so as to be able to use their wisdom.

Oriental & Occidental Philosophies

The use of needles in order to ease some health problems within the body is known as acupuncture. It is an accepted practice in both Eastern and Western medicine.

In Western medicine it is used to treat postoperative pain, as an alternative to anaesthesia, to treat menstrual cramps and many other disorders. The needles are used to stimulate many points in the body which are selected carefully to deal with an exact symptom or a set of symptoms. Insertion of needles may have no sensation or may cause a warm and pleasing sensation to flood through the body. It also helps a patient relax and the results are fast because pain is relieved quickly.

Explanation of its working principle comes from China wherein the inhabitants of this country have practiced acupuncture for over two thousand years. Hence according to the Eastern philosophy, the body works properly when the vital energy travels around the body as it is meant to. The body then said to be in balance between two diverse principles namely Yin and Yang. To enhance understanding, the former is associated with relaxed, cool and passive objects and feelings and the latter is indicative of warm, active and assertive objects and actions.

Energy flows from one organ to another, balancing Yin and Yang. This energy is known as Qi and in the event when it might have been blocked or reduced, the body is unwell and begins to manifest symptoms. It is Qi that is believed to control the physical, mental, emotional and spiritual aspects of a human being.

An acupuncture practitioner treats depression, anxiety and other emotional issues with as much flair and confidence as treating physical symptoms, owing to the theory that Qi, regulates the human body. Certain symptoms that are a cocktail of physical, mental and emotional issues are also due to imbalance of Qi and can be treated with acupuncture. This is why specific questions are asked pertaining to the history of a patient to determine the diagnosis and treatment does not solely rest on physical symptoms.

Study of the effects of acupuncture has been of interest in Western medicine for the past twenty years and there has been a great success in its usage during this time. Finding an explanation for the results through Western medicine only is baffling owing to the manner in which the problem is addressed. The explanation as of present is that, the needles influence the nervous system and stimulate it into producing biochemicals which in turn produce a positive effect in treating the symptoms. How the stimulation is created is a point that requires further investigation. Other studies show that acupuncture alters the brain chemistry, thus affecting functions of the body in the process.

Whatever the explanations may be it must be said that the field is interesting and needs to be explored more thoroughly. It is relatively new from the research point of view and future advances will not only render explanation of its mechanism simpler but also promote understanding of its underlying principle.

Variations in Techniques

The picture a person generally envisions in his or her mind about acupuncture is that of a person seated on a chair with needles protruding out of his or her skin in several parts of the body. Indeed acupuncture does entail the use of needles to help regulate energy flow in certain areas of the body with the intention of eliminating various health conditions.

In acupuncture, needles are inserted in to a certain depth of the skin and are usually more close to the surface. However, the needles could be inserted to a further depth, depending on the treatment being administered to a person. These could be left in place for a short duration of about thirty minutes or for longer periods and can even be twirled in place, warmed before insertion or heated during insertion. There is no discomfort except for a slight pinch felt sometimes, which is not often. Relaxation, slight warmth or even a rush of energy may be experienced during treatment. Some may feel nothing at all. Whatever the feeling is, it must be understood that the treatment leads to the change in the symptoms of a person after a period of time.

Certain variations of acupuncture are used that do not call for the use of needles. The principle of understanding of the acupuncture points, organization of the body and the importance of the accurate energy flow throughout the body is basic to the standard acupuncture technique. However, the difference is that certain other techniques are used to stimulate the acupuncture points and needles are omitted altogether.

One such technique is sonopuncture. It is a device that produces sound waves to be applied to a point where a needle would have normally been inserted. Apart from this, devices that cause vibrations such as a tuning fork could also be used. The results have not yet been established as is the case with the needle based technique.

Application of a low voltage electric current to the acupuncture point is another technique which was used for some time. This is done together with the insertion of the needle or by touching a wire connected with a low voltage of electric current to the surface of the skin. The feeling is a light tingling but not a painful sensation. This technique was developed independently in America and Europe in the 1930s and 1940s, but it seems that the interest in this area dissipated after that period.

Another technique which is a variation of acupuncture is the use of acupressure. No instrument is used in this case and instead pressure is created by pressing on the acupuncture point with the finger. The technique can be integrated to certain other techniques such as shiatsu massage. By looking at a diagram which has the pressure points of the hands and feet, even a lay person is able to perform the technique. However for it to be effective the person should have an understanding of the whole system of acupuncture and not just the location of the acupuncture points.

Apart from the above, friction, magnets, suction and even laser beams have been thought as being instrumental for being used in acupuncture treatment. Acupuncture on the whole is a great method to bring back the balance of the human body.

Human Organs and Acupuncture

Most people visit the acupuncture clinic, not being cognizant with the principle underlying the technique. The acupuncture practitioner however possesses vast knowledge of the subject, allowing a person to be treated effectively.

A normal person identifies the organ system of the body as individual units but in Chinese medicine and in Eastern medicine the organs are viewed similarly and yet differently. Every organ as seen with both views is meant to perform a clear cut function of the body. In Chinese medicine however, each of these organs carry an internal energy known as Qi and certain pathways that this energy uses to flow throughout the body are known as meridians. Each organ generates a great amount of energy during certain times of the day and at certain times the activity declines. Therefore according to this ancient system the organ is not just a structure but it is like a structure-energy parcel that controls the behaviour and supports a person to go on living.

To Chinese medicine twelve organs are important. These include the stomach, heart, kidney, lung and liver. These are important when dealing with Western medicine as well. However Chinese medicine further segregates them - the small and the large intestine are two separate organs and the pericardium or the sac around the heart is also a separate organ. The gall bladder and urinary bladder are important and are considered as separate organs, but these organs are not as important in Western medicine as in Chinese medicine. There is the identification of another organ in Chinese medicine, known as the "triple warmer" organ, which is particularly replete with Qi energy and is a set at three locations in the torso.

These organs are important because that a healthy body and mind is due to the normal flow of Qi in acupuncture. Therefore knowing the locations of these organs and the flow of Qi energy in and around them is vital in reconstituting the normal flow. Certain symptoms have been associated with certain abnormalities of a particular organ. For example dizziness, rib pain and blurred vision imply liver dysfunction. By physical observation and by taking the history of physical, mental and emotional issues from the patient the organs affected can be determined and treatment carried out.

Acupuncture stimulates Qi using needles and restores the flow of energy. If an organ has a deficiency of Qi, another organ known as a donor organ will be assigned to supply the energy to the deficit organ, hence implying the importance of energy flow between the organs. Therefore a certain amount of treatment using acupuncture ensures energy flow in and around an organ, showing improvement in one or many symptoms.

The actual mechanism that governs the success of the treatment using acupuncture is an area that yet has to be explored. However getting to know about it through the available information could prove to be very interesting and would also help to keep health in check.

Diagnosis by a Practitioner

Acupuncture deals with the usage of needles to address certain health issues. This is done by the needles being used for redirecting and balancing the force in the body, known as "Qi", When a person undergoes physical, mental and emotional problems it is due to this energy or Qi being out of balance at one or more points in the body.

The diagnosis is done very differently as compared to a typical Western style of diagnosis. In such a situation the practitioner takes the pulse of a person by holding both the wrists. The pulse is observed at several different points, not just one and this is then evaluated. After this, the points as to where the needles should be inserted are then decided. These should be placed at certain strategic points that are thought to be the best to tackle the issue.

When taking a person's pulse there are several factors that a practitioner is on the look-out for. Up to 12 different pulse points of a person can be taken. Three surface pulse points and three deep pulse points are taken from each wrist. Depending on the depth and location wherein these pulse readings are taken from, even an untrained person can notice the differences. Six of the common pulse descriptions in acupuncture are floating, sunken, slow, rapid, slippery and choppy and an acupuncturist should be adept enough to distinguish between them.

Observing the tongue of a person is a useful technique for diagnosis. Even Western physicians are able to diagnose a throat problem by observing the coating on the tongue, but an acupuncture practitioner looks for many other symptoms. For an experienced acupuncturist, the tongue of a person can narrate its own tale and he can piece together the riddle of the illness by observing aspects like the color of the tongue, both top and sides, cracks and swelling on the surface, state of the dots and the amount of moisture. These provide an insight on the person's health and point out what the treatment plan should deal with.

Western medical diagnosis is not of much help in acupuncture. In acupuncture a particular diagnosis may be an outcome of one or many different interruptions in the flow of energy or Qi. This is why the diagnosis of Western medicine is of no value. It should be kept in mind that each symptom should be described in detail. Taking pain as an example, the time the symptoms are most severe and the time that they are less severe, if it reduces after a good night's rest should be described.

An acupuncture practitioner does not look just at a symptom, rather he or she looks at the way a person's organs and system interact and find out which one provides a clue to the existing symptom. This in turn leads to finding the perfect treatment option for a person opting for this traditional form of treatment. Therefore anyone considering acupuncture should not be surprised to find that the clinic of an acupuncture practitioner different from a normal clinic of a Western medical practitioner.

Acupuncture Needles

Acupuncture deals with restoring the energy circulating through the body to its usual levels. In order to ensure this, needles are inserted at certain points on the skin, which are determined by the practitioner in accordance with the person's symptoms which could be emotional, physical, behavioural and mental.

The needle inserted at these points regulates energy by either increasing or reducing it. Energy is increased by acupuncture in case there is a reduction in its levels at certain points, as is shown by the symptoms of dizziness or depression. Energy is reduced by acupuncture, if there is an excess at certain points, as is shown by symptoms of heat or anger.

By analysing a person's symptoms the organs involved with the symptoms are determined. This in turn decides the points which the needles should be inserted at. There are different types of needles in use and several types of techniques used to insert them. Small, disposable needles are available for use nowadays and these are inserted at different depths according to the symptoms shown by a person. The techniques used to stimulate or increase energy is different to the techniques used to dissipate or reduce energy. Exactly how it is done definitely makes interesting reading.

Needles used to stimulate energy produce better results when warmed. The point of insertion is massaged before insertion and then the needle is inserted to the correct depth slowly, with superficial puncturing of the skin. It has to be removed slowly as well. Insertion is carried out when the person exhales and extraction occurs as the person inhales. The points are punctured according to energy flow and the needles are left up to ten minutes at these points.

Prior to insertion, the needle used to dissipate energy is not warmed, is inserted and removed promptly, leaving it in the skin only for a few seconds. These needles are inserted at more depth. The points are punctured in the opposite order from energy flow. The needles are inserted as the person inhales and removed when the person exhales. This technique used to dissipate energy can be compared to letting air out of a balloon and like a balloon releases air, the person also exhales when the needle is removed, thus releasing energy.

There is no pain when the practitioner inserts the needle. The first insertion may have a feeling of a slight pinch but this is not a common occurrence because henceforth the needles are hardly felt and the patient quickly forgets about them. There are several different needles, however the patient cannot tell the difference unless it is a Japanese needle. Japanese needles are different because these come in a guide tube and are thinner. Needles are of different widths as well and those that are used for dissipating energy are definitely thicker than the ones used for stimulating energy.

Indeed the using of needles is fascinating when discussing about acupuncture. If anyone is considering acupuncture, he or she should go ahead and do it without being frightened that needles are being used, because the needles do not hurt a person in any way during the process.

How Many Sessions Will It Take?

More and more people are showing an inclination towards acupuncture these days and some traditional physicians even refer patients to acupuncture clinics simply because acupuncture addresses symptoms much more effectively and without side effects. Acupuncture is used to treat symptoms relating to pain, emotional distress and many other physical, mental and emotional conditions.

Symptoms, age of the person, length the condition existed and the environment the person lives in are factors that decide as to how long the treatment should last. Some patients are more responsive than others to the treatment and hence may need only one or two sessions. This is seen most often in children. Adults who show a better response generally require one to six sessions in order to experience results. Certain others may require up to twenty visits to control their symptoms. Some rare cases such as recovery from paralysis may also take place after years of treatment. Hence it is seen that the length of treatment differs from person to person.

Some conditions require daily treatment. Conditions such as chronic pain need daily treatment until the pain subsides and application of acupuncture to stop drug abuse requires daily treatment to help keep the desire at bay. In some cases, the first session of treatment may have a noticeable improvement, while subsequent sessions may show aggravated results while in other cases, the first treatment alone may aggravate the symptoms. Such results should be brought to the attention of the practitioner who will sometimes modify the position of the needles.

Acupuncture has a marked effect on headaches, head congestion, cramps, be it menstrual, muscular or intestinal, all kinds of pain, depression, fatigue, haemorrhoids and nervous disorders in children. In the case of diarrhoea, painful menstruation, eczema, gastric problems, kidney and gall bladder dysfunctions, nervous disorders, palpitations, rheumatism, shingles, autonomic nervous problems following surgery, acupuncture has some rate of success, but not as significant as the ones specified above.

New areas that acupuncture is successful are coming into light and hence if someone has a condition other than those that appear above, it is good to consult an acupuncture practitioner. Acupuncture is thought to help alleviate symptoms caused due to tuberculosis, infantile paralysis and Parkinson's disease, rather than cure the disease itself. It is surprising that in some instances acupuncture has been successful when traditional medication had failed. Take a look at the following examples.

A woman suffered with pain in her ankle for three years and in spite of having tried standard medication her agony remained as bad as ever if not worse. An experienced acupuncture practitioner observed her symptoms carefully and cured her in three sessions. Likewise, a farmer was suffering from low grade fever (fever of around 100^0F) every night for several months. While normal physicians could not even determine the cause, an acupuncture practitioner administered regular treatment to no effect. The practitioner then changed the time of day to treat him to very early in the morning and his fever disappeared completely.

These are just two cases out of the very many cases of success. It may sound like a miracle to some suffering from certain chronic disorders for long periods of time. Therefore if someone is considering acupuncture as a treatment option it will be a great idea to try it out.

A Visit to a Clinic

Acupuncture is considered as a remedy for many health-related issues such as constant pain, stress and weight loss. In China, where acupuncture originated, people use it as a method to maintain a healthy body. The acupuncture practitioner in China gets paid only if the client does not fall ill and maintains a picture of good health throughout. But before taking the plunge learning more about this method of treatment is strongly recommended. The adage 'Look before you leap' comes to mind here and gaining an insight as to what happens in an acupuncture clinic and what one looks like in America is certainly reassuring.

Even though the clinic typically looks like an office, modus operandi of diagnosis is different and occurs in two parts. The first is a physical examination and the second is a discussion of the symptoms and the environment in which the patient spends most of his time. Physical examination is carried out by closely analyzing the tongue and taking a reading of pulse. Unlike in normal Western medicine, the pulse reading is taken of both wrists and on various points on each wrist, both near the surface and deep below the surface. The observations are then duly noted.

During the discussion, if it is a first visit, focus would be mostly on the symptoms. The patient should have a clear picture about the symptoms and be able to tell the practitioner about these in great detail. For instance if the pain is in the ankle, the patient should be aware of what causes the severity of pain to increase and decrease. It could be the time of day, certain activities like walking or standing for a great period of time or a certain time of year or month. Stress could also one of the factors that could lead to pain. Possibility of pain ensuing due to a new supervisor at work or any other emotional issue should also be explored so that all physical, emotional and social aspects that may have an impact on a symptom are covered.

At the end of the discussion all points are taken in to consideration and the initial diagnosis is made and subsequently a treatment plan is then chalked out. Treatment may commence on the first day or the patient may be given an appointment on a different day to return in order to begin treatment. The specific day and time of administering treatment is important for it to take effect.

Treatment session lasts for less than an hour. Very thin needles are inserted at specific locations, decided by the practitioner and for a certain amount of time according to the person's symptoms. Insertion and removal of needles are usually painless - however there may be a feeling of a slight pinch, like the bite of an insect, which disappears quickly. During the session the patient may feel nothing, may feel more relaxed, or feel an increase in energy or a warm sensation at the points of needle insertion. The basic purpose of the needles is to regulate and rebalance circulation throughout the body no matter what the initial feeling might be.

These visits should be enjoyed, owing to the knowledge that acupuncture ensures restoration of health to its normal state.

Using Herbs with Acupuncture Treatment

When thinking about acupuncture, the first picture that comes to mind is that of a person sitting on a chair with numerous little needles sticking out from various parts of his or her body. This is correct to a great extent although the needles used are very thin and are confined only to a certain area and not everywhere as one would imagine.

Our body comprises of a certain energy that has to be in balance to ensure its proper functioning. Quite often the balance of this energy is disturbed due to various internal and external factors. This is when the body is said to be "sick". Needles used in acupuncture help to balance this energy and this in turn leads to recuperation from whatever the ailment it might have been suffering. The degree of treatment required to bring back the balance depends on the person and the symptoms that he or she is manifesting.

Acupuncture as a form of treatment began in China thousands of years ago and since it was a part of traditional Chinese medicine, herbs have always been a part of treatment. These herbs are specific for the symptoms a person is being treated for and may be in form of pills or capsules or could be taken as a tea, brewed in warm water. Not all herbs are used and the only the appropriate herbs meant for a particular set of symptoms are mixed and given. The proportion can also be adjusted if several different herbs have to be used and the action is rapid as the herbs are taken in form of tea. Raw herbs which have the most potency can be prescribed. However the taste of raw herbs may not agree with a person who is not accustomed to the idea but once it is taken several times a person gets used to the taste and the issue is resolved.

Not all acupuncture treatments deal with the administration of herbs because even without them the treatment is effective. A practitioner should be informed beforehand if any nutritional or vitamin supplement is taken by a person, such as garlic pills, if herbs are been introduced in the treatment. The reason for this is that sometimes these supplements may interact with the herbs given. Also it is advisable to inform about any prescription medication taken by a person.

It is imperative to inform the practitioner if a new symptom comes up after herbs are administered. While it is normal to have a slight upset in the digestive system, but if even this or a symptom different to this is noticed the practitioner should be notified. Therefore herbs can provide rapid relief to a symptom and enhance recovery but it is not an essential component in acupuncture treatment.

Treatment for Women's Issues

Acupuncture is used to control pain, relieve stress and deal with other emotional problems. It has also proved effective in treating problems pertaining to women's health such as menstruation and infertility. Each individual has a different set of problems and an acupuncture practitioner can address the problem of each patient specifically. By going through some of the case studies where the issues were rectified with the use of acupuncture, an individual can form an unbiased opinion of this treatment method.

The first case is of a woman with painful and irregular menstruation – the lady was depressed and irritable and displayed frequent bouts of anger. Her pain increased when she was angry. If looked closely it was evident that there was an association with the cause which is menstruation, the symptoms which are physical as she experiences pain, mental as she is irritable and emotional as she gets angry. The correlation between, the increased intensity of the pain when she is angry is also a point which is noteworthy.

An acupuncture practitioner asks questions that address all four areas and a patient should be vigilant to give a detailed description about the symptoms. On being analysed, the symptoms point out that anger and irritability is due to energy trapped in some organ or area of the body. Menstrual irregularity also when taken to account hint that the organ that should be addressed is the liver. Several consultations with the acupuncture practitioner helped resolve the emotional correlation with her menstruation and also the pain accompanying it.

In the second case, the lady in question was in the stage of menopause. She experienced hot flashes and pain in the lower back. The acupuncture practitioner discussed about the energy around the kidney. As we grow older the energy in the kidney reduces which leads to the ceasing of menstruation. This energy is normally in balance, the two ends of see-saw being Yin and Yang. Hot flashes indicate an increase in Yang and as she experienced pain in her lower back, it suggested that increase in energy because Yang is located in the kidney. Acupuncture treatment was then targeted at the kidney, to rebalance the energy around it. With this the symptoms disappeared.

Then there was the third case of a thirty-six year old woman who could not conceive. Standard Western methods used for testing revealed her hormone levels to be normal, but yet she was unable to conceive. She had an irregular menstrual cycle and was depressed and because this was similar to the first case and indeed treatment targeting the liver was started. In this case too treatment targeting the kidney was included because as was seen with the second case, the energy in and around the kidney is what regulates the menstrual cycle. The problem of her not conceiving could be addressed only after her cycle was regulated. Owing to the gravity of the condition this patient required more than a few sessions recover show improvement.

By this it could be seen that acupuncture can be used to treat certain issues relating to women's health. It is only a method that uses needles in its treatment and a person does not have to be afraid as no medication is administered.

Acupuncture to Look Beautiful

Some of the common problems that acupuncture helps to overcome are pain, anxiety and stress relief. As results are positive, more and more people are opting for this ancient Chinese method of treatment. However how many people are aware of the fact that acupuncture can be used in beauty culture also?

There are many people who stare at the mirror every morning before applying makeup, wishing that the fine lines, dark circles under the eyes and pores would go away. Some women who are might be ageing wish that that hint of a double chin and age spots could be got rid of. In order to remove these some go to the extent of plastic surgery and even consider using Botox. Well, it is indeed possible to overcome all these problems by using acupuncture. A few needles used in acupuncture are much easier to tolerate than having to undergo plastic surgery. The tiny needles in acupuncture treatment when inserted into the skin of the face stimulate the production of collagen in the particular area which in turn stretches out the fine lines and wrinkles.

Results have been noticed with a few sittings of acupuncture procedure. Not only does the complexion clear and gives a glow to the face, wrinkles and fine lines also become less prominent. All that the treatment does is to bring the energy of the face to normal and keep the face in a healthy state. After the face is cleared the attention then can be focused on the rest of the body, starting with weight loss.

So many people try to lose weight through exercising, regular visits to the gym, embarking on diet plans and yet do not find the required results. It has been virtually impossible to maintain an attractive waist and hip size no matter how hard a person tries. Acupuncture has proved to have an answer to this annoying problem. Unlike many of the weight loss regimes that promise the moon and fail to deliver even the earth, acupuncture is a time-tested and effective technique.

This is also done by the use of needles. Thin needles are inserted into various parts of the body in order to redirect the energy and keep the body in functioning appropriately. Inclusion of herbs or herbal tea in the diet is also recommended alongside treatment. According to Western scientists, the treatment is successful due to the discharge of the chemical endorphin. It is this chemical that helps a person to lose weight. After losing weight to the desired extent, treatment is then administered to maintain this weight.

Paying a visit to the acupuncture practitioner on a regular basis is definitely recommended to help balance the energy of the body. It is a course of action that will help a person keep healthy, stay in good shape and look beautiful for many long years to come.

Acupuncture During Pregnancy

To always hope for the best for the baby is the very essence of motherhood and while this process commences at conception it continues throughout the life of the mother. Caring for a baby by its mother begins long before the baby is born. A mother who is expecting a baby is very cautious about what she eats and how and when she should exercise. It is to this effect that some expectant mothers now have begun to seek acupuncture treatments. Normally being once a month and lasting for around forty five minutes, in the ninth month the frequency of treatment is increased to weekly to prepare the mother for labour.

Acupuncture has been known to reduce the duration and intensity of morning sickness of an expecting mother during the first trimester. During the second trimester, heart burn is a common complication. With acupuncture this can be reduced to a great extent. Oedema and high blood pressure which are sometimes seen in pregnant women can also be reduced with acupuncture, but the physician should also be consulted before hand as these could be a warning about other major complications. During the last trimester back and joint aches are the common complaints. Acupuncture can rectify these issues and align the baby in preparation for delivery.

Regular treatments help to eliminate toxins effectively and keep the mother in the best of her health during pregnancy. The womb environment is kept balanced, helping the baby grow and thrive and minimize complications that may arise during pregnancy. It can also be used to induce labour in a woman who is overdue. When acupuncture is used in inducing labour, the woman feels relaxed and warm, the reason being the reduction of stress and anxiety which is of great benefit. This is opposed to the feeling a woman gets when oxytocin is used to induce labour. The energy of a woman is also enhanced during labour with acupuncture.

Acupuncture can be used post delivery to stop a woman from bleeding. Insertion of a needle at the acupuncture point will help stop the blood flow. Acupuncture injections for several weeks after delivery could help reduce post-partum depression and anxiety that a woman may feel subsequent to delivery and help the body recover rapidly to regain its normal state.

Midwives nowadays are been trained in acupuncture techniques. Acupuncture practitioners should undertake certification programs in most American states and women who consider acupuncture during pregnancy should look for this certification. More often acupuncture treatment is teamed up with herbal medication for optimum results. Therefore certification is issued for the usage of herbs as well. This certification should also be considered if both methods are been used.

Acupuncture is proving to be a great method for a pregnant mother to find relief. A certified practitioner and trained midwife pave the way for both mother and baby to have a great start together in their journey of life.

Acupuncture and Electricity

Pain, stress and a variety of diseases are some of the health conditions that have been successfully treated through the application of acupuncture. One possible technique of method of treatment entails applying a tiny electrical charge to the needle. The use of low levels of electricity in medical treatments was limited to the 1930s and 1940s, but has recently begun owing to increasing interest in this form of therapy.

Acupuncture was developed over centuries by careful observation of tenderness in specific points that accompanied the manifested symptoms. It works on the principle that energy is evenly distributed and continually flows through the body. If energy levels are depleted or concentrated at a point, the disruption causes disease or discomfort. Acupuncture helps to restore the correct flow and distribution of energy from concentrated points to depleted points. This is accomplished, very simply, by inserting needles into the skin of the client.

Success of the treatment depends on the point at which the needle is inserted, as also the depth and the technique employed. Different techniques include applying heat, also known as moxa, using herbs, either separately or at the site of insertion and applying a low voltage electrical charge to the acupuncture points instead of inserting a needle. The nature of cells dictates that they are electrically charged. When that charge is disturbed, the electrical properties of that point are altered. Using

Kirlian photography, we can observe the effects of this energy because the shape of the energy before an acupuncture needle is inserted is different from the shape of the energy after the needle is inserted.

Scientists using infrared photography have been able to observe the temperature variation between acupuncture points and the skin that surrounds them. Their findings support the fact that the electrical properties of acupuncture points behave differently to those of the surrounding tissue when the patient is suffering from a certain symptom. Thus scientists using electrical apparatus were able to discover and duplicate the acupuncture points discovered centuries ago.

Other electrical research also seems to support the principles behind acupuncture. Fractured bones have healed much quicker than they normally would when treated with a low intensity electrical pulses. This seems to validate the experiences of clients who have received beneficial acupuncture treatments for broken bones in the arms, wrists, feet, ankles and elsewhere. Becker is a scientist who has successfully grown healthy tissue in animals by the application of a low-level electrical current to the damaged tissue. Even the tissue of the heart has been repaired completely and devoid of all scarring.

Likewise, acupuncture is known to be effective in the treatment of patients suffering from heart palpitations. This has been recorded by an EKG machine which is attached to the patient throughout the duration of the acupuncture treatment. Something that was apparent was a structural change in the heartbeat, which is dictated by electrical impulses received from the nerves.

Thus acupuncture and electricity are intricately connected already. Add to that the experiments that were conducted during the 1930s and 1940s, as well as the recent research, and the result is an exciting field of research in acupuncture. Therefore, in addition to herbs, electricity is another form of acupuncture treatment.

Acupuncture and Drug Abuse

For a drug addict or alcoholic the compulsion to find one more fix or have one more drink is sometimes irresistible. These compulsions can be both physical and psychological. If the recovering addict can deny the compulsion, then one more successful day is possible.

There are chemicals that can help ease the withdrawal symptoms, such as nicotine patches for those habitual smokers. However, acupuncture is another avenue for recovering drug addicts and alcoholics. There are a number of advantages of acupuncture treatment for addictions. The main advantage of using this method is that there are no chemicals involved. Apart from this, it is also relatively well priced in comparison to other treatments for addiction and withdrawal. Also, acupuncture is not specific to one kind of addiction and can treat a wide range of different addictions.

The question may occur - what effect does acupuncture have on a recovering addict? First you need to understand the compulsion that an addict experiences when they feel that they have to have another fix or another drink as soon as possible. Acupuncture creates a physical change and is often described as relieving that compulsion, like taking off your shoes after a tiring day on your feet. This effect only lasts for a day however. Addicts who have only started recovering will need to undergo sessions every day.

Dry alcoholics and others who have been recovering for a longer period of time only need to get a treatment occasionally, when they feel they need it. This can be only rarely, when they encounter stress due to problems in the home or work environment. An acupuncture clinic is extremely beneficial in times such as these when that compulsion once again becomes unbearable.

Consider a rehabilitation clinic that employs acupuncture as a treatment for addiction. The setting is rowdy and unpleasant before acupuncture was introduced, but now the atmosphere is tranquil and serene in spite of as many as five patients, who can be quite unsettled. The room where the patients receive their acupuncture treatments accommodates a large number of chairs arranged so that patients can see each other and interact during while the session is in progress.

This helps ease new clients who may be wary of this technique. The needles are placed in various positions, depending on the specific needs of each client, and remain in place for about forty-five minutes. All treatment methods involve five needles in each ear and some may have additional needles in feet, arms or hands. These are removed after the recommended time by the acupuncture practitioner, an assistant or the client themselves.

There are a number of such rehabilitation clinics and acupuncture treatments are the initial steps for each patient. A ten day schedule with daily acupuncture treatments and tests, to ensure that the patient has not used any drugs in the previous day, starts the program. After the first ten days of being "clean", the patient is then able to begin other therapies, like a twelve step program, while continuing with the acupuncture treatments. In the event of a relapse, the patient would need to start from the beginning with the ten day acupuncture treatment.

Acupuncture used in a rehabilitation program is economically, physically and mentally advantageous for addicts in recovery. This is one more example of how acupuncture heals the person as a whole in every aspect.

Acupuncture and Children

All parents would want their children to enjoy a life of health and happiness. It is worth considering treating the health of your child through acupuncture. Not only is acupuncture a curative treatment for a variety of ailments, but it is also used as a preventive measure. In fact, some acupuncture practitioners in China are only paid while their clients are healthy.

Do children really go for acupuncture treatments? Surprisingly, yes. In fact, children generally feel that acupuncture treatments are painless and even pleasant. They tend to be more in tune with their bodies than adults are and because of this they can feel the treatment working to make them well again. Although the basic treatment remains the same for children, in terms of the best time for treatment and the points of insertion of the needles, they generally do not need as many sessions or needles for treatment. This is because their bodies are very active and not as much stimulation is needed for a quicker and more remarkable improvement. A child can get acupuncture to remain healthy as well as to approach a physical ailment or for problems in behavior.

Children do not have the negative association with needles that adults do, and the younger they are, the more it holds true. Inserting acupuncture needles is not painful and unless they are moved, they cannot be felt after they have been inserted. Maximum that can be felt is a slight pinch when the needle is inserted, but typically not even that can be sensed. The needles can be inserted just under the skin or as deep as a few inches and the depth depends on the treatment requirements.

Ultimately the aim of acupuncture is to treat the person as a whole and bring the physical, mental, emotional and social aspects together harmoniously. In order to do this a number of factors need to be taken into consideration. Physical symptoms like pulse and the condition of the tongue are taken into account as well as behavioral indicators like depression, anger or aggression. Even the time of year and the external environment of the child are considered.

A problem seen quite often is that of bedwetting. For some children, only one session is needed, while others need a couple more. Parents often notice the negative emotions of the child and automatically conclude that it is a result of the bedwetting. After some consideration however, they realize that there was an emotion or unhappiness that came as much as a few weeks before the bedwetting began. Although it is not always true, there is generally a preceding cause and not just the child feeling bad about wetting the bed. Focusing this attention on the child as a whole greatly benefits the entire family as well as the child.

Another concern to consult with your acupuncture practitioner is childhood vaccinations. The number of diseases that can be vaccinated against is constantly growing. Chicken pox vaccine, for example, has been growing in popularity. Not all of them are necessary, but your acupuncture practitioner may have a number of vaccines that he will advocate, like the polio vaccine, and it may be worth discussing in detail. You should view your acupuncture practitioner as a general health specialist for your child.

Acupuncture and Biorhythm

We are all affected by biorhythms. The way the position of the sun changes throughout the day and the particular position of the moon throughout the month both influence the way our internal clocks regulate our bodies. This is evident in the effect on our bodies in response to minor adjustments like daylight savings time and even more evident in the effect on our bodies to major adjustments like jet lag. In addition to the twenty-four hour cycle, there are also cycles that span ten days and they are affected by the moon.

In the last three or four decades the Western world has become more aware of biorhythms and our understanding continues to grow, along with our interest. However, the ancient Chinese were well aware of how our bodies are intricately connected with the position of the planets and have been applying their knowledge to their practice of acupuncture for centuries.

The energy of our body fluctuates in response to these biorhythms, with every organ experiencing a period of the highest energy output as well as a period of the lowest energy output. Each of these two periods spans two hours for each organ and the order in which the organs experience their maximum energy outputs forms cycles throughout the body. In correct order of this cycle, first is the liver, followed by the lungs, then large intestine, then stomach, spleen, heart, and so on for each of the twelve major organs. When the energy is highest, the symptoms affecting that organ are the worst. This is also the best time to treat the symptoms.

Symptoms experienced by the person can help an acupuncture practitioner to pinpoint the organs and energy channels that are affected. One symptom may indicate too much energy while another indicates too little. Details of these symptoms and their associated organs and energy levels have been recorded in numerous books. An organ with too much energy should be treated during the time of its maximum energy while an organ with symptoms of energy deficit should be treated immediately after the time of maximum energy. When it is not possible to make an appointment with your acupuncture practitioner during these times, there are other times of the day that are almost as good to undergo treatment.

It is the ten-day lunar cycle that may make a particular day best for the treatment of a specific symptom. This is because there are two aspects of the Qi energy as well as five elements. Each day in the ten-day cycle is associated with a different combination of the elements with the Qi energy aspects. Each organ is coupled with a specific element and so treatment would be more effective on days linked to that element.

In order for treatment to be most effective, it is imperative that the timing of the symptoms and the exact symptoms are recorded. It is also important to realize that the times and dates of the treatments are a vital component of the treatment itself.

Stress, High Blood Pressure, and Acupuncture

A stress response in the body occurs when certain chemicals are released as a reaction to stress. These chemicals cause the heart rate to increase, the breathing to become more rapid and the muscles to become tense. This is excellent if the person is being hunted by a vicious predator, but if the person happens to be a businessman negotiating a particularly stressful deal, then this reaction does him no good.

Occasional bouts of stress are dealt with by the body with ease as the chemicals are cleared from the system and the muscles relax. If this stress response is experienced on a regular basis, like a few times a week, the resting state of the body becomes affected. The muscles are unable to completely relax and the chemicals that are released cause other problems like troubled sleep, stomach and digestive problems, panic attacks and pain such as headaches. Continued stress over a long period time can cause more severe problems such as strokes, high blood pressure, colitis, or other bowel problems.

There are a number of things that can hide the effects of stress and some people believe that they are managing their stress with such aids, but they offer only temporary relief. For example alcohol, caffeine, cigarettes, sugar or even antidepressants prescribed by a physician. Even though prescription medications can help with the psychological and physical effects of stress, they don't eliminate the reason for the stress. Often that is not an option, which is when acupuncture can really help.

Acupuncture works on eliminating the effects of stress from the body, first by relaxing the client and then by removing the tension in the body. Relaxation results in a drop in the heart rate, lowering of the blood pressure and an increase in energy and even to regenerate damaged tissue. The energy in the body is stimulated and redirected where it is needed so that every muscle, every organ and every system can function properly. This leaves the client feeling healthy and confident. Many times acupuncture has eliminated the need for a prescription antidepressant in addition to relieving the stress. If acupuncture were used by more people with stress the American population would be a lot healthier and we may even see a dramatic decrease in prescription drugs like Prozac.

Although the standard technique of using acupuncture needles is extremely effective for the treatment of chronic stress, it has been found that using low levels of electricity in conjunction with the acupuncture treatment allows the blood pressure to be lowered more successfully. Researchers have shown that mild electrical stimulation has been proven to grow healthy tissue to replace damaged tissue in animals without additional scarring. Combining acupuncture treatments designed to manage blood pressure with the possibility of growing healthy tissue is an exciting prospect for people with heart and circulatory problems.

Stress is a problem for most Americans and acupuncture is among the most effective treatments for it. With the use of acupuncture, the symptoms are reduced and the health of the whole body is improved.

Acupuncture and Extreme Cases

Acupuncture has a wide range of different uses. There are even some extreme examples when acupuncture can help where modern medicine cannot. Here are just a few of these examples.

The first possible case where acupuncture can help is when a person is in a coma. At a time when my father was receiving treatment in a hospital for long term care, there were two patients who were in comas. One of these had been in the same condition for months and to my knowledge had not received any visitors. The only help the hospital could give was basic care, essentially taking care of him until he awoke from the coma. There is not much a doctor can do after they have treated all the symptoms they know of.

This is where acupuncture comes in. While western medicine classifies patients in a coma by the cause of their coma, such as a brain tumor or car accident, acupuncture bases treatment on the symptoms that are shared. By inserting needles at specific points, the energy in certain organs will be redirected and help to clear the physical senses, quiet the patient's spirit, clear the mind, make the heart stronger, and get rid of phlegm. In some patients the needles may even be gently rotated. These acupuncture treatments improve the patient's general health. Sometimes, although medically we are unsure as to why, patients will awake from their comas.

In the second extreme case, acupuncture is useful is for patients who faint regularly. After a physician has eliminated major heart problems as a possible cause, acupuncture can be used. Some standard acupuncture treatments can restore the circulation of blood to the whole body, which includes the head. If the fainting is caused by a social problem like working too hard, or an emotional one like wanting to escape from a certain situation, acupuncture will help those too. In this way acupuncture heals the physical and emotional aspects, thus treating the patient as a whole.

Acupuncture is valuable in emergencies. Although the best option would be to have an acupuncture practitioner immediately available in the event of an emergency, this is not usually possible. Here are some straightforward techniques that can be performed by anyone. In the event of a patient losing consciousness there is an acupuncture point that could cause them to wake up. This point is in the furrow between the nose and the mouth and can be found approximately one third of the way down from the nose. A firm force should be applied with a fingernail. There is an acupuncture point that can help with ailments involving the chest such as palpitations, hiccups, stomach pain, and lung problems. In such cases, press firmly on the underside of the forearm and approximately two thumb widths from the last crease of the wrist. This point is between two tendons.

These are only a few of the cases in which acupuncture could help. There are other methods that could help patients who were drowning and are not yet conscious but are breathing, people who are in shock, people with broken bones, and many more. Hopefully this selection has helped to expand your mind about the possible uses of acupuncture.

A Personal Experience

Imagine that Susan is about to venture into the hitherto unknown area of acupuncture for the first time. All she can think about is having dozens of needles sticking out of her in every direction, from strange places, until she is unable to sit anymore. When she told her friend Marie about the problems she has been experiencing with depression and trouble sleeping, Marie recommended the acupuncture clinic she had been going to.

Marie did not seem like the type of person who would do anything this unusual. She appeared to be incredibly healthy, regularly exercising at the gym while still having plenty of energy afterwards. But apparently this was not always the case. A few years ago Marie went to her family physician with severe cramping. Her doctor suggested that acupuncture may give her partial or complete relief from the cramps. The treatment made Marie feel so much better and after going to the clinic she found out that many people get acupuncture treatments regularly to maintain good health. Since then Marie has been getting regular treatments for, as she puts it, "tune ups". Susan was amazed to find out that Marie would ever visit an acupuncture clinic, let alone keep going for more than three years. Even more amazing to Susan was that a physician would recommend it.

This is the first treatment session that Susan has ever received in the acupuncture clinic but it is not the first visit. Her first consultation with the acupuncture practitioner involved a lengthy discussion of the symptoms she was experiencing along with number of her vital signs. At this consultation Susan related the relief she was hoping to get from her depression and trouble sleeping through the acupuncture treatments. There was a surprising amount of questions that she had never considered before. For instance, was the sleeplessness identical every night or were some nights more restful than others? Or was it easy to fall asleep again after waking up in the night? Now that it was spring, the central heating in the house was turned off and Susan could not remember if the sleep trouble started before or after that change. She had to answer a number of questions about that. There were also an unexpected number of questions relating to her depression.

Her work environment had changed when her best friend found another job and that could be related to her depression. She was also asked about any previous depressions that she may have experienced and if she had noticed any pattern emerging. After she had answered all the questions, the acupuncture practitioner recommended that she make an appointment to have her first treatment on a different day for the best possible outcome.

So today was that day and Susan was still slightly anxious when she parked in the parking lot, in spite of the fact that the acupuncturist was a lovely, calm lady. After twenty minutes Susan found herself seated in a comfortable chair with possibly eighteen needles inserted on a number of points over her arms and ears. The needles did not hurt and Susan found that she was most at ease. After about fifteen minutes the acupuncturist returned and removed the needles. Once the recommended treatment schedule, comprising six sessions, had been completed they would reassess Susan's symptoms. Susan was surprised and pleased that it had been so easy.

Yin and Yang and Acupuncture

Harmony can be described as a perpetual balance of opposites. In ancient China it was thought to be the ultimate state of being, as a person and as a society. Acupuncture is used to restore harmony when there is a disruption in either the physical or emotional characteristics of the person.

There are opposites in everything, from colors to energy and actions. While the Chinese gave them distinct poles, namely Yin and Yang, Western society denotes these same concepts as positives and negatives like ions in chemistry and physics. Yin and Yang are not in opposition with each other, rather they represent the extremes of each given spectrum. A bit of both is needed for harmony to prevail. For example Yin is rest, cold, winter, quiet and passive while Yang is active, hot, summer, volatile and antagonistic. Nothing can exist completely as one extreme. When these opposites are out of balance, the harmony is disrupted. This causes the flow of Qi, or energy, to be constricted or overemphasized at different points in the body.

Acupuncture seeks to restore a state of harmony to the person as a whole and thus considers the physical state as well as the mental and emotional states. In order to assess a client, the acupuncture practitioner takes note of any imbalances on four sets of features. While the first three sets are specifically for hot vs. cold, interior vs. exterior and excesses vs. deficiencies, the fourth set is a general feature that is not covered by the first three sets. As an example, consider an unusually passive person who spends the majority of his life indoors and eats a lot of sweets. This person will have two specific imbalances - inside and excess and extremely passive.

A disharmony may not necessarily cause physical symptoms. Problems with the family, crying easily and other problems involving the emotions or socializing may indicate the presence of an imbalance. The Qi energy is constantly in motion. If the flow is disrupted the acupuncture practitioner can determine where the disruption is by the specific symptoms. For example, an accumulation of energy in a certain point or organ could result in the client becoming overly aggressive and easily angered. Alternatively, an energy deficiency in a given point or organ may cause the client to become depressed and experience lack of vigor. Taking this into account, along with the physical symptoms, allows the acupuncture practitioner to devise the best treatment in order to optimize the flow of Qi and restore balance to the person, physically and emotionally.

Essentially the acupuncture practitioner uses the "Yin" and "Yang" extremes to examine the items, activities, environment and any other aspects in the life of the client. With these results the problems can be more easily identified, whether they are mental, social, physical or emotional, and the appropriate treatment schedule for each individual can be drawn up. The practitioner then uses acupuncture to re-establish the proper flow of Qi through the body and that returns the client to a state of balance and harmony.

Acceptance in America

Acupuncture has been gaining popularity in the United States over the past two or three decades. The most remarkable and successful uses were for reducing pain or eliminating it altogether. There are even cases where a patient has undergone a surgical procedure with no anesthetic, using only acupuncture needles to eliminate pain. Acupuncture is a technique that was first developed in China and Japan and has been in use for centuries and it is courtesy of Jesuit missionaries that it was introduced in Europe during the 1700s'.

Currently, over ten million U.S. adults are using acupuncture or have used it before. This number does not include children, but acupuncture is entirely safe for them. Quite often children respond more readily to acupuncture treatments and obtain better results than adults. The use of acupuncture as a method of relief from pain or other symptoms is growing among health practitioners. Thousands of traditional physicians, dentists and other medical professionals are supporting the use of acupuncture.

Because of the growing popularity of acupuncture in a medical setting, National Institute of Health has become interested in it and has held numerous conferences focusing mainly on the use of acupuncture. Designing a study that leads to unquestionable results is very difficult. Because of this there are ongoing debates about the success of some of the studies that have been done on acupuncture and its efficacy in relieving a given group of symptoms.

In general, however, it is agreed that acupuncture gives effective relief from numerous symptoms such as post operative pain and nausea, headaches, asthma, osteoarthritis and menstrual cramps, to name a few. Studies are ongoing and more results are being published regularly. The best way to keep up with the studies is to search the Internet using the particular symptom you are interested in, together with the word "acupuncture" as key words. The National Institute of Health has a branch that investigates alternative medicine called NCCAM. Websites sponsored by this branch are the most reliable.

The main equipment used by an acupuncturist is specialized needles. In order to guarantee the safety of these needles in an acupuncture office, they need to be regulated by the government. The FDA has approved the use of these needles in acupuncture clinics by practitioners who are fully licensed in their use. The needles are required to be sterile and used only once to prevent needle contamination, similar to the needles used in a traditional medical setting. The acupuncture practitioner should use a new, unopened package of needles for each patient and the site of insertion should be prepared by swabbing the area with a disinfectant such as alcohol.

Acupuncture has become an established practice with credit given to it by both the medical community as well as government institutions. Acupuncture is not only recommended by doctors.

Many have even become trained in the technique themselves. Acupuncture clinics and practitioners are government regulated through standards of practice to guarantee the safety of the patients. Thus, although it originated in China, acupuncture has been accepted as a part of the American health system.

The American Academy of Medical Acupuncture

Some people may be surprised to learn that an increasing number of medical professionals advocate acupuncture as a valid treatment, and some even practice it themselves.

Almost twenty years ago, a number of physicians trained in acupuncture wanted to promote the use of it in regular medical practice, and so they founded the American Academy of Medical Acupuncture, or the AAMA. The AAMA sets high standards for its members, including the traditional medical practitioners as well as certified acupuncture practitioners. This allows the patient to have absolute confidence in the training and standards of practice of their practitioners.

In the past there was a clear division between acupuncture and western medicine. Acupuncture practitioners were well versed in the philosophy and techniques behind the practice of acupuncture, but knew very little, if anything, about western medicine. On the other side of the divide, western physicians had no knowledge of traditional Chinese medicine and were highly suspicious of the claims of healing that acupuncture made. This divide is now narrowed down considerably.

There have been numerous studies and experiments proving the efficacy of acupuncture in healing certain symptoms, like persistent pain. In some cases, physicians began trusting the care of their patients to the techniques of acupuncture practitioners. Some physicians eventually learnt the history and techniques of acupuncture in order to integrate these techniques into their own treatments. The UCLA School of Medicine played a big role in this by sponsoring courses.

The AAMA is devoted to increasing the understanding and acceptance of acupuncture by medical professionals and other physicians who are currently unaware of its benefits. Most physicians are aware of the possibility of using acupuncture in place of anesthetic during operations. Acupuncture is also being acknowledged for its use in a post operative setting to reduce pain and nausea. In addition to this, acupuncture also has numerous possible uses in an emergency room.

Research is among the top priorities of the AAMA. Researchers of interest to the AAMA are those who study the applications of acupuncture that are new in medical settings, be it a hospital or a physician's office. Particularly interesting to the AAMA is research into the reasons of why acupuncture is as effective as it is. This is because a lot of physicians want to understand the process set in motion by inserting needles into certain points and why those points are significant. A lot of research has gone into explaining these mechanisms.

Results are submitted to the magazine published by the AAMA called Medical Acupuncture. This journal integrates western medical knowledge with traditional and modern techniques of acupuncture through the use of medical papers, case reports and research results. The efficacy and safety of acupuncture in many areas such as cancer, gastroenterology, strokes, urology, pulmonology, pain relief, and OB/GYN is explained in the journal as well.

The number of certified physicians trained in acupuncture is growing. Because of this we can be sure that patients will benefit from both areas of expertise and the general health of America can only improve.

Finding a Practitioner

Given the surge in popularity of acupuncture as a method of treatment, it is but natural for any individual suffering from a medical issue to opt for it. Feeling ill could probably be described as being one of the worst states of mind for any person and that is why people often do not leave any stone unturned in their attempt to regain good health. While it is true that Western medicine does have answers to many questions, alternatives like acupuncture can also be explored simply because of their balancing techniques.

For anyone who wishes to embark on an acupuncture treatment, the journey would begin by embarking on a quest for an acupuncture practitioner. In this era of computers, Internet is the first search option that comes to mind and all that is required is typing in of a few appropriate keywords to acquire a list of physicians in that area. Word-of-mouth references can also be sought from friends, relatives and known physicians as there might be someone who might have opted for this mode of treatment before. A personal discussion also serves to abate many fears because acupuncture is a branch that is often shrouded with many baseless myths and misconceptions.

Having prepared a list of acupuncturists in the area, it is time to check on each one of them in order to establish their veracity. Amongst the several parameters, the foremost pertains to certification and although a certificate is just a piece of paper, it is an assurance in itself that the particular physician has undergone formal training. Making inquiries pertaining to the type of training undergone by the acupuncturist and their background in the field is a must while trying to make a choice. For example, no-one in their right mind would put themselves in the hands of a dentist or a surgeon who is unable to show any documents verifying his qualification.

Identification of an acupuncturist is a process that may be time consuming but still worthy because it would not only ensure cognizance of the problem but also speedy recovery. After checking on all the names on the list and eliminating ones which may not have survived the scrutiny, it is time to establish contact with the selected few and adjudging their quality of treatment through their response. Calling up and talking to them on phone is indeed more convenient but a strong recommendation would be to pay a visit to their office to assess their professionalism.

Comfort is an imperative factor while finalizing an acupuncturist because it is one of the seminal determinants of the success of treatment. Unless a patient feels completely at ease with the physician not just while discussing the symptoms but also during the sessions, the outcome of the treatment will not be positive. Last but not the least will be the cost of treatment and this would be worked out only after all the discussion and chalking out of the entire treatment schedule. Charges would vary from one physician to another and comparison shopping is the way to go in order to find the best possible deal.

An important point that needs to be borne in mind is the fact that owing to its roots in ancient Chinese medicine, acupuncture is more concerned with treating the symptoms rather than pinpointing the disease. Therefore, curative though it might be, this method should not be relied upon to seek a specific diagnosis but just to restore the body's energy flow for long term good health and well being.

www.ingramcontent.com/pod-product-compliance
Lightning Source LLC
Chambersburg PA
CBHW070609290526
45790CB00002B/848